Healthcare communication

Healthcare communication

A rhetorical handbook

Patrick Muller, M.A.

Writers Club Press
San Jose New York Lincoln Shanghai

Healthcare communication
A rhetorical handbook

Writers Club Press
an imprint of iUniverse.com, Inc.

For information address:
iUniverse.com, Inc.
5220 S 16th, Ste. 200
Lincoln, NE 68512
www.iuniverse.com

ISBN: 0-595-19974-7

Printed in the United States of America

DEDICATION

This volume is dedicated to my teachers.

Henrietta Logan, Ph.D.
    University of Florida

Sandra Schuldt, M.A.T.
    University of Iowa

The Rev. Susanne Watson
    Iowa City Free Medical Clinic

Linda Yanney, Ph.D.
    Iowa City Free Medical Clinic

Jane Rowat, R.D.H., M.S.
    University of Iowa

Kay Mescher, R.D.H., M.S.
    University of Iowa

and Dr. Marcy Rosenbaum, Jeannie Panther, Dr. Kristi Ferguson, Dr. Geordie Lowry, Dr. Don Brown, Bill Radl, Ted Nelson, John Lynch, Yvonne Wernimont, Dr. Ginny Woodard, Dr. Eric Evans, Dr. Paul Hottel, Dr. Nyle Kauffman, Dr. Ozzie Diaz-Duque, Dr. Teresa Marshall,

Prof. Marsha Cunningham, Prof. Jamie Sharp, Dr. Al Bolden, Dr. Howard Field, Dr. Steve Levy, Dr. Cathy Watkins, Dr. Mike Finkelstein, Mary Kiritsy, Dr. Jed Hand, Dr. Ray Kuthy, Dr. Yolanda Edwards, Dr. Chris Anderson, Dr. Chris M. Anderson, Dr. Mike Ross, Dr. Todd DeBoom, Dr. Aaron Bossler, Clarence Haverkamp, Harriet Tripp, Larry Hertel, Steve Carlson, Ric Graf, Ed Arensdorf, Mary and Barbara and Sandy and Christine at the Iowa City Free Medical Clinic, Lori Ziegenhorn, Dr. John Leupold, Dr. Kyle Talbot, Dr. Howard Cowen, Dr. Marcia Boyer, Jane Jakobsen, Dr. Shadi Chamany, Dr. David Goodwin, Dr. Loraine Frost, Dr. Meryl Severson III, Dr. Chris Bauman, Dr. Matt Casey, Dr. Matt Larson, Dr. Matt Jensen, Dr. Jeff Moser, Dr. Kaleo Staszkow, Dr. Robert Doty, Pauline Taylor, Marjorie Caruth, Dr. Mickey Eliason, Dr. Deb Liddell, Dr. Al Hood, Dr. Bill Matthes, Dr. Kay Coangelo, Dr. Ernie Pascarella, Dr. Leslie Baxter, Dr. Dennis Maki, Dr. Ursula Delworth, Dr. David Bills, Dr. Steve Desjardins, Dr. Bob Engel, Dr. Mary Trachsel, Dr. Brad Sagen, Billie Townsend, Dr. Peter Densen, Dr. Christine McCarthy, Dr. Scott McNabb, Dr. Al Henkin, Dr. Lelia Helms, Dr. Takis Poulakos, Dr. Fred Antczak, Dr. Les Margolin, Dr. Joyce Moore, Dr. David Depew, Bonnie Bender, Pat Zousel, Tina Craig, Prof. Tess Judge-Ellis, Dr. Stacie Walton and Lisa Santiago.

for m.s.

Contents

Healthcare communication

Iowa City
First draft; August 2001
Comments, suggestions, and corrections are welcome and encouraged.

A Rhetorical approach to healthcare communication

What is Rhetoric?

In common parlance, rhetoric is thought of as political "spin," opinion, verbal sleight of hand, exaggerated argument, or even an untruth. "There they go again, giving us more of their rhetoric. We give you the truth." In academic circles rhetoric is misunderstood as well. There is a focus on rhetoric as the study of argument and persuasion. Since examination of the argument or persuasion, however, rarely includes an examination of and an evidential defense of the underlying values system—for example, often the reason- and order-biased Western tradition—arguments are not really examined; only opinions are examined.

[Rhetoricians who cannot step outside of their own value system and critique an argument from a meta-(transvalue) perspective are not really evaluating an argument and thus truth. They are merely evaluating a jockeying of opinions.]

Human beings make sense of the shape of the world they encounter and actually reshape the world they encounter through language. The patterns they use to ascribe meaning to the world and the stories and portraits they have of themselves and others, these language-based activities shape the human world. Rhetoric is the study of these language-based activities.

In the vernacular, Rhetoric is the study of lines, stories, and voices. What lines are drawn; where; and by whom? What stories are told and by whom? What voices are heard and taken seriously; what voices are heard and mocked; and what voices are silenced? And then, how does all this posturing affect the truth and reality that people live?

Why a rhetorical approach to healthcare communication?

Philip Phenix, in *Realms of Meaning*, broke knowledge into nine domains. A revision of his model shows at least sixteen ways of knowing: anthropology, art, economics, education, history, law, medicine and healthcare, philosophy, physical education, political science, psychology, science, sociology, and ultimate concern. Many of these ways of knowing—especially economics, law, medicine, science, and ultimate concern—like to claim that their way of knowing equals truth. None of these ways of knowing equals truth. All of these ways of knowing are templates or models with algorithms (theories, interventions) that allow us to access truth.

Rhetoric is a way of knowing. Rhetoric is about drawing lines, using language, and recognizing voices. Since patient-centered healthcare is ultimately about knowing where the patient and clinician draw the lines; knowing how the patient and clinician use language to modify their worlds; and having an awareness as to what voices are privileged and what voices are silenced in the healthcare setting, the discipline of Rhetoric has a lot to offer a patient-centered approach to healthcare.

Theology is a subset of ultimate concern: the human quest to find meaning, to matter, to belong, and to continue in some fashion. Religion is ubiquitously and inappropriately trumpeted as the sole vehicle to ultimate concern. There are many other vehicles.

Some common misconceptions about Healthcare Communication

I've been babbling since birth and communicating even before that. I know how to talk to people.

In the conversations we have with people we tend to avoid negative responses. When we ask someone how they are, we expect them to say, "Fine." Unless patients present themselves for a wellness check, ultimately, they will say they are NOT fine.

We routinely do not ask strangers or even friends about pathology, alcohol use, substance use, sexuality, sexual activity, and sexually transmitted diseases. We ask patients about these things all the time.

We never ask a stranger we've just met if we may stick a finger in one of their body orifices. Dentists, dental hygienists, dental assistants, and other team members ask this question routinely. We never ask—no insist—that a stranger takes off his or her clothes so that we may gawk at and/or fondle hi or her body*, particularly their genitalia, but physicians, nurses, and other team members do this all the time.

The conversations you will have with patients and the requests you will make of your patients, you have little, if any, experience. You have not been communicating like this since birth. Odds are you have not ever communicated like that.

*You would, I know, prefer words like inspect, examine, palpate. You say Po-Tay-to; I say Po-Tot-o. In the end, no matter how you slice it, you are gawking and fondling.

I agree that communication is important; however, you are either born with the talent or not. I am not a natural. Therefore I just have to make do. I cannot be taught this.

Granted based upon your cultural or individual responses you may feel comfortable or non-threatened asking potentially sensitive questions about sexuality, substance use, and so on because you have less hangups about the body, sexuality, and substance use. You may have had a more heterogeneous life experience than most.

Even so, communication skills can be taught. You can follow a template that will make this communication more effective. And this template can be taught.

Men are from Mars; women are from Venus

Human beings have a proclivity to find patterns to organize and make sense of their world. One persistent and inaccurate pattern in which we find ourselves is this notion of mutual exclusivity of gender.

Research shows that everyone uses both sides of their brain and deploys both reason and emotion in sustaining a functional personality. In fact, it is when one side of your brain or your ability to reason or emote is incapacitated that your personality can suffer dramatic dysfunction. Intragender differences are far more varied then intergender differences. And we won't even get into here the parts of sex, gender, and sexual orientation that are socially constructed.

We carry around these stories in our heads that males are leaders, assertive, the political animal, of reason, independent, and left-brained. We say to ourselves that females are followers, nurturing, the domestic animal, of emotion, connected, and right-brained. Again, the reason/emotion and right/left stuff do not hold up as well under scrutiny as our stories would predict. In addition the brain is rewirable. Your brain is being rewired just by reading this. By the time you are done reading this booklet you will physiologically be a slightly different person. But even if you do have a physical proclivity for reason or emotion, what does that say? Like every human being, in any capacity, you use what you have; you make do; and you constantly adjust. If you are 5'4" or 6'0", those are "immutable" physical characteristics. In some instances, being 5'4" may enhance your life experience—for instance, when sitting in a movie seat with little leg room. In some instances, being 5'4" may impede your life experience—for instance, when examining a really tall patient. You may have to use a step stool, lower the exam table, or try some other strategy. The point is we constantly make adjustments for "immutable" physical characteristics as we go through our day of work and leisure. But we don't make these physical characteristics problematic and stereotypical the way we do with genitalia. If you don't make genitalia problematic, then Mars and Venus aren't quite as distinguishable as you claim.

Research was conducted. Put men—the reasoned, independent, and assertive ones—in an environment where they were expected to be and the stories (mythology) affirmed them to be more nurturing and they became markedly more nurturing. Put women—the emotional, connected, and nurturing ones—in an environment where they were expected to be and the stories affirmed them to be more assertive and they became markedly more assertive. So John Gray has found a nice pot of gold peddling his wares. It turns out, however, that if the mythology allows and affirms it, men and women both are from Mars and Venus, to some extent.

And what about the binaric and inaccurate conversation we have about men and women that we haven't address yet. These are the conversations that men are the political creatures and the leaders and that women are the domestic creatures and the followers. If you believe these culturally constructed truths, how does this affect you if you are male and your professor or chief resident is female? If you believe these culturally constructed truths and you are female, how do you become team leader, an authority to the patient—especially a male one, a professor, or a chief resident?

Isn't this talk about voices and cultural construction overblown?

We have these notions in society that men are not supposed to cry, be emotional, show vulnerability or compromise, be afraid, or have pain. Now that more women are stepping into the political (traditionally in this culture the masculine) arena, more women are subjected to those expectations. We wear hats that say "No fear" and we run around the gym chanting "No pain, no gain." We have a preponderant and repugnant attitude toward these things; and yet pathology and disease and even wellness checks can present all of these things in a patient. Do you have an inaccurate conversation in your head that emotion, crying, vulnerability, compromise, fear, and admittance of pain are moral infractions? And if so, how does that impede the care you provide your patients?

What is the number one prescribed therapy in all of healthcare? Rest. And do we live in a (capitalistic society (that eradicated the southern European tradition of siesta) that values action or rest? Many men and many women participate in athletics at some point in their lives. What are some of the biggest mantras heard from the coaches? Play through your pain. If you are not succeeding, punch it out. In other words, the strategy for failure or lack of growth is more practice, more action. Action, action, action. Do you have a love affair with action? And does that love affair impede the therapy you provide? Do you see a patient who cannot play through pain or who cannot suck it up and tough it out to be a moral transgressor?

The culturally constructed conversations we carry around in our heads can greatly affect how we view and interact with our patients. We need to have a greater understanding of culturally constructed conversations and we need to be more aware as to how they can impact our patient interaction and care.

What we need is cultural competence.

A noble, but unattainable, goal. Individual identities (sex, gender, sexual orientation, race, ethnicity, age, political affiliation, ultimate concern) and human cultures are confluences of biology, language, mythology, environment, history, and contingency. Identities and cultures are none of the things we claim: original, pure, static, concrete, mutually exclusive, and simple. Identities and cultures are paradoxical: originally interactive, purely hybrid, staticly fluid, concretely confluential, exclusively overlapping, and simply complex.

Since it is the mechanism of the brain's physiology and a culture's strategy to legitimate itself to categorize, stereotype, and so on to eliminate the richness for the sake of function, we are shut out to most of our possibilities. Think of the things you didn't like as a child—that you said were not and would not ever be a part of you—broccoli, spinach, classical music—that you like now. Imagine the things that you don't like now, that someday you will cherich. My contention is that you do not even know yourself, so how could you know any other?

And your knowledge of cultures is not any more impressive than your knowledge of individuals. Cultures are not phenomena of truth or possibility as much as they are agents of conformity. When you say you know your culture, you are saying you know what are the dominant expectations to which people are expected to conform that manifest themselves in mythology, ritual, artifacts, institutions, and relationships. You do not at all know how people would interact or appear if they didn't have to con-form to this set of stories. My contention is that you do not even know your own culture, so how could you competently know any other?

This makes sense. Colin Powell is an AFRICAN-American. Do you think he in any way has the same life experience, predicated on African-Americanness, as an uninsured, poorly educated African-American factory worker in Georgia? Do you think he has the same life experience as an African villager living in fear of the next time a harsh wind brings the Ebola virus sweeping down the river valley? An upper-middle class, col-lege-educated, health insured, and resident of a gated community white person has as much, if not more, in common with Colin Powell that this African-American factory worker in Georgia.

Since identities and cultures are composed and recomposed from dynamic confluences of they constantly change. It is impossible to know—be culturally competent—in any identity or culture, including one's own.

It is, however, possible to be culturally competent in knowing the con-fluential mechanisms that make up identities and cultures. It is possible to be competent with the sensitivity that your patients, Colin Powell and another the black factory worker from Georgia, do not necessarily share the same stereotypical racial or ethnic experience. It is possible to be aware that every patient filters identity and culture through his or her own per-sonal experience and interactions. You are always treating an individual; you are always less so—many times much, much less so—treating a repre-sentative of any type of cohort. Cultural stereotypes may be instructive as guidelines to locate the general vicinity of your patient's background or makeup; they never fix your patient in a specific locale.

Reality is the same for everyone.

"I was clear on what transpired to the exam and I was clear about the instructions. The patient even said there were no questions. So how could the patient now say things happened differently?"

It seems reality is the same enough for us in some broader veins. For instance, if the appointment is in Clinic A in the South Wing at 11 a.m., the clinician and patient will both show up in the same physical space at approximately the same time. But what happens during that encounter? What patient and clinician will take from that encounter will be based not as much on the facts but on their responses to the facts. Our responses to the facts are going to be filtered through our unique and dynamic confluence of biology, language, mythology, environment, history, contingency, and experience.

So, yes, patient and clinician will experience the same physical space but not necessarily the same encounter. This makes communication—an attempt to gauge the patient's perceptions and interpretations—even more essential.

Rapport is just small talk

Even incidental, "small," talk can be shown to build relationships and enhance more significant dialogue. But the way rapport will be defined here as many more important implications than "just shootin' the breeze."

Healthcare communication, especially rapport, is a luxury and, in these times of managed care, an insane waste of time.

Have you heard of the 15-33 Rule? It is a phrase I coined from doing research on healthcare communication. Clinicians who do or do not engage in patient-centered healthcare communication have a profound affect on their patients' well-being.

Communicative patient-centered clinicians:

- accelerate healing
- decrease the frequency and
  intensity of relapse
- decrease morbidity

These positive effects are likely due to greater compliance and continuity of care engendered by such communication.

Clinicians who eschew patient-centered communication:

- decelerate healing
- increase the frequency and
    intensity of relapse
- increase morbidity

These adverse effects are likely do to reduced compliance and disconti-nuity of care engendered by such communication.

Patients seem to consciously or inherently sense this. Clinicians who practice patient-centered communication experience a 15% turnover in their patient pool. Clinicians who do not practice patient-centered communication experience a 33% turnover in their patient pool.

Clinicians who use patient-centered communication get sued less. Patients who received patient-centered communication sue less.

So if clinicians do not want to learn and practice patient-centered communication for a noble reason: providing optimum patient care; they may do so for more crass economic reasons: less work needs to go into drumming up new patients and less time and money is loss to defense in law suits.

HEALTHCARE RAPPORT

The patient-centered healthcare template presented in this handbook will be based upon Interview Rapport. Two types of rapport will be discussed: upfront rapport and conversational rapport.

 For a more descriptive discussion and as a complement to this text, please visit the following website:

bailiwick.lib.uiowa.edu/healthcare-rapport

What can rapport do for the patient and me?

Many generalists I've talked to say they can make a diagnosis 40-60% of the time just by talking to the patients. Some specialists I've talked to say they can make a diagnosis 50-80% of the time just by talking to the patient. But just as clinicians immediately start assessing patients when they encounter them so do patients assess clinicians. Patients will not "spill their guts" to anyone wearing a white or blue coat. Patients come to healthcare professionals seeking help, often because they feel compromised. A patient's first task, always, is to protect himself or herself. If a patient feels that giving information to the clinician may cause the clinician to think poorly of the patient, discriminate against the patient, or put the patient in harm's way (for instance, informing an adolescent patient's intolerant parent of the patient's drug use or sexual activitity), the patient is more likely to withhold, distort, or minimalize that information which may impede diagnosis and thus therapy.

Clinicians may want to pay attention to rapport for several reasons.

Rapport builds trust. Taking interest in the patient's world and getting to know something about the patient's world builds trust. Trust increases the forthrightness of the information the patient gives. Trust increases compliance and continuity of care.

Rapport builds relationship. Rapport builds the relationship that happens later in the appointment. This increases compliance. Rapport builds the comfort level of the patient, so the patient may return to this clinician for care.

Rapport quickens diagnosis. Rapport enhances communication and forthrightness of patient's information. Thus diagnosis is accelerated.

Rapport builds a practice. Rapport builds relationship. The patient returns to the clinician's practice and is not part of the annual turnover. The patient refers family, friends, associates, and even strangers to the clinician.

Rapport gives a window onto how the patient communicates and processes information. This knowledge can be used to enhance future encounters, diagnoses, and compliance.

Rapport is important for a couple other reasons.

We do not know when a patient will next have contact with the health-care system. Even if a patient has traditionally been a regular seeker of care, this patient may drop out. So any preventive or education or relationship-building efforts spent in this appointment, which rapport will certainly enhance, may be invaluable to this patient. Especially efforts that go beyond one's clinical expertise or the matter at hand. An opthamologist who notices a questionable mole or listens when the patient remarks she hasn't been to the dentist in five years and suggests the patient go see a dermatologist (or her physician) or a dentist may be doing the patient an invaluable favor.

You may be the clinician the patient most trusts. So even though you are the patient's physical therapist, when you suggest the patient go see a dentist, the patient does so. When the patient's physician suggests this, it falls on deaf ears.

A RAPPORT TEMPLATE

As we begin to look at rapport and healthcare communication using a more systematic model, let me point out several themes that runs through all of this.

We cannot ever know the patient, his or her identity, and his or her culture. We only get glimpses of the patient and we can only make stereotypic, distorted assumptions about the patient's identities and cultures. All your straight patients are not carbon-copies. All your African-American patients are not carbon copies. All your male patients are not carbon copies. All your First Nation patients are not carbon copies. All your lesbian patients are not carbon copies. All your 15-year-old patients are not carbon copies. All your European-American patients are not carbon copies. All your bisexual patients are not carbon copies. All your Latino patients are not carbon copies. All your 80-year-old patients are not carbon copies. All your Christian patients are not carbon copies. All your female patients are not carbon copies. All your Pagan patients are not carbon copies. All your Shinto patients are not carbon copies. All your Jain patients are not carbon copies. All your agnostic patients are not carbon copies. All your Jewish patients are not carbon copies. All your Muslim patients are not carbon copies. All your Ba'hai patients are not carbon copies. All your Buddhist patients are not carbon copies. All your atheist patients are not carbon copies. All your Confusician patients are not carbon copies. All your Latina patients are not carbon copies. Are your Asian-American patients are not carbon copies. All your gay patients are not carbon copies. Colin Powell is not the same African-American patient sitting before you as the high school drop out, uninsured, factory worker from rural Georgia. You can, however, get to know something about the patient's world by asking open, inclusive, patient-centered questions. The best cultural competence you can achieve is not on the identity or cultural level but on the patient level. Even with the same patient, every encounter is different. You change over time and context; the patient changes over time and context. The patient may reveal some aspects of self and community in one encounter, for whatever reason, than in another. Having an awareness of the dynamic multifactedness of the person on your exam table or in your operatory and being somehow sensitive to that complex being in front of you is perhaps the best and most appropriate cultural competence you can achieve.

Every question or statement from you is an invitation or a denial for the patient to open up and tell you things about himself or herself. You want to create those invitations frequently throughout the appointment. You do this with open, inclusive questions.

You want to keep this encounter a conversation and partnership rather than an interrogation and dictatorship. You do this by asking umbrella questions.

Some thoughts on questions

Every question (and statement) you ask frames reality and sends messages. Open, inclusive, and umbrella questions help you frame reality and send messages in ways that you might want the patient to receive them.

Leading question. Coerces the patient towards in answer. Tells the patient what you want to hear, so the patient will often give you that. Useful in summarization; possibly harmless in small talk. A waste of time or distorting elsewhere. "You brush your teeth twice a day, don't you?" "You understand these directions, don't you?" What do you want your patient to say to such questions? You've already given your opinion on which—yes or no—is the "better" answer. But is it the accurate answer.

Closed question. Usually answered by one word with no elaboration. Good question for clarifying or ascertaining specific information. It focuses and closes down conversation into one area, so this question is not good for general probing.

Open question. Usually encourages a lengthy patient response, though the patient can shut it down with a closed response. (For example, what have you been up to this summer? Not much) Non-ideal question for gathering specific information quickly. Ideal for general probing and relationship building.

Inclusive question. You can only assume you know the patient's world. And the patient will give you what you give the patient. Ask a male patient if he likes sports. If he does, he will say yes, and you may talk about sports at length. But you haven't ascertained anything about the complex individual sitting before you. You've just laid out a socially constructed expectation, assumption, and/or conformity for the patient and he has met it. If the patient does not care for sports, then you've put the patient in an awkward position, which may cause the patient to start to detach from you. It will take more energy to explain his world to you, who thinks the world must revolve around sports, then is actually worth it. So this patient may also talk about sports or just shut down. Since we can not ever know a patient's likes or dislikes, why not just let the patient tell us himself or herself by asking inclusive questions.

Framing reality. Every question you ask takes us in a certain direction and frames our answers. If you ask me what my favorite ice cream is, vanilla or pralines-and-cream or chubby hubby is an appropriate response. If you ask me what my favorite sport is, then tennis or triathlons or gymnastics is an appropriate response. But you would think it rather silly or strange if you asked what my favorite sport was and I said vanilla. So the questions you ask frame what I can talk about and thus frames our conversation and thus our reality for the next few minutes. If you always ask me about sports and then we always talk about gymnastics, then you might get the impression that I am a big gymnastics fan, which is moderately true. But you might also get the impression that gymnastics is the center of my world, which is definitely not true. You would say to others, "Yeah, gymnastics, that's all he ever talks about." To which I would clarify, "That's because sports is all you ever ask about." Sometimes a patient will tell you something much later or tell someone else a different angle on a story. You will think, how come you never told me that? To which the patient is likely to respond, because you never asked and because you never gave me the opportunity to tell you.

The way you can guard against the former—you never asked—is to ask open, inclusive questions. The way you can guard against the latter—you never gave me the opportunity—is to ask umbrella questions.

Umbrella question. This is really "the kitchen sink" question. "Tell me your story." "Tell me about yourself." "Tell me more about that." "What else would you like to tell me about your health?" "What else would you like to tell me about this pain?" "What other questions do you have?" "What else would you like to discuss with me today?" Variations on these types of questions allow the patient to contribute information or question you in ways that they feel are appropriate. If you keep asking about the patient's headache or aching tooth, where does he or she throw in information about swollen ankles or bleeding gums or a concern about a family history of diabetes or an interest in orthodontic work? Since you cannot possibly know what are all the right questions to ask or what all the patient's possible concerns or interests are, don't waste time trying to guess or assume. Ask an umbrella question and give the patient a chance to tell you.

UPFRONT RAPPORT

Spend a couple minutes, even 30 seconds, getting to know the patient. Get or confirm residence, daily routine, hobbies, and relationships. If you ask about these things in an open, inclusive manner, you will establish some trust, build a relationship, enhance and quicken diagnosis, all by getting a sense of the patient's world and creating a safe, nonjudgmental space for the patient to talk. Knowing something about the patient makes it easier to ask more sensitive questions later on.

What are some good ways to initiate a conversation?

If the patient is cogent and not under duress—for a first visit or wellness check—"tell me about yourself" is a good kind of opening. If the patient is under duress, some of the following can be ascertained "on the fly."

Asking a patient how they would like to be called or deferring to the formal, until the patient instructs you otherwise, is better than asking, "Would you like to be called Mr. Sinnwell or Adrian?" With that exclusive question, you've only given the patient two choices—YOUR choices. The patient may not like either one or feel you are forcing him into the familiar (Adrian) or feel like you are making him seem stodgy if he answers, "Mr. Sinnwell." Try not to put the patient in that position.

In addition to asking for whom to notify in case of emergency—on a form or in person—ask a patient—on a form and/or in person—if there is someone special he or she likes to discuss important medical decisions with. Leaving it open like that allows the patient to answer a relative or a partner. (A potentially harmful way of asking a patient is to ask a female if she wants to share medical decisions with her husband when she may be single, going through a divorce, widowed, in a partnership with a man but not married, in a partnership or marriage with a woman, or in a polyamoric relationship.) This is a good way to inquire about relationship.

Why would I want to know about residence (geography) for diagnostic and therapeutic reasons?

"I see you are from Forest City; where is that in Iowa?"
 "What kind of a town is Forest City?"
 "How long is the drive?"
 "Did you come alone?"
 "Did you have any trouble finding the clinic?"

These types of questions can give you a sense of escorts (and relationships) and transportation. You will may want to know about ease or difficulty in getting to the clinic for further appointments. Is the patient able to drive or take the bus? Does the patient have his or her own transportation? Does the patient rely on a ride—personal or commercial? Will today's or a future procedure necessitate an escort for the patient? You may get a sense of relationships from this conversation. You may want to know more about relationships later on.

Distance from clinic will be significant in scheduling future appointments. Will the patient be coming with someone else who would like to coordinate an appointment as well?

Why would I want to know about residence (structure) for diagnostic and therapeutic reasons?

"Do you live in a house or apartment?"
  "Do you have flouridated water?"
  "Do you live alone or with someone?"
  "Do you have any pets?"

Maybe the patient's chief complaint is environmental. Maybe the house has radon or carbon monoxide poisoning. Maybe the chief complaint (flu, cold, food poisoning, absetous poisoning, lead poisoning) was passed from or shared with an infected/affected housemate. If no one else in the house is having these symptoms, then it is likely not carbon monoxide poisoning.

Why would I want to know about someone's daily routine for diagnosis and therapy?

Occupation could be the source of one's chief complaint (occupational injury, stress, environmental exposure to toxin). Occupation will also play into scheduling future appointments and continuity of care. If you only perform a certain procedure/treatment on Mondays and Wednesdays and it is difficult for the patient to get time off on those days, then the patient may stop seeking care.

If someone needs to change a dressing or apply eye drops every so many hours, how might they do that at work? If you recommend a patient stay home from work the next four days but the patient only has two days of sick leave left, what therapy can you recommend that would induce healing and not get the patient fired?

What are ways to ask about someone's daily routine?

Asking someone "where do you work?" or "what kind of work do you do?" could possibly leave out and offend a homemaker or the unemployed. While you cannot avoid offending people entirely, when you can see in advance that something might be exclusive, it might be best to avoid it.

Try asking "what do you do?" or "if you didn't have to visit the clinic today, what would you normally be doing?"

Why would I want to know about hobbies for diagnosis and therapy?

For many of the same reasons you want to know about occupation.

While most people think of hobbies as a source of pleasure and well-being, they could be a source of illness. Overspending on a hobby (gambling, expensive adult "toys") may blow the patient or family's budget, thereby inducing stress. A painter could expose himself to toxic chemicals. A carpenter or computer fanatic may induce carpal tunnel syndrome from her leisure activities. A hiker or camper's illness may be tickborne. Knowing the patient likes to camp or hike may quicken diagnosis.

Exercise is often recommended as a therapy. Knowing a patient likes to bike, the recommended exercise therapy could be tailored to a bicycling regimen.

Good ways to ask

What do you like to do for fun?

So when you are not busy being a dental, medical, nursing, pharmacy, physical therapy, physician's assistant student, what do you like to do to kick back and relax?

Why would I want to know about relationships for diagnosis and therapy?

Significant others, work associates, friends, and housemates can be sources of stress, infection, and abuse.

Often questions are framed in relation to housemates. "Did everyone else eat the chicken last night? Is anyone else sick?" "Does anyone else in your household have these symptoms?" "Do you find you are hot and turning down the thermostat while everyone else in the house is running for a sweater?"

Significant others, friends, and housemates may also be caregivers. "This dressing needs to be changed twice a day. Do you have any one at home who can help you with that?" "After the operation you won't be able to drive the car or lift more than 5 pound items. Will someone else be able to drive the kids to school, do laundry and go grocery shopping?" Relationships can play in important factor in healing and wellness.

Significant others, friends, and housemates may need to conform to the patient's patterns even if they do not have the same diagnosis. For instance, the household starts drinking skim milk instead of two percent because skim is what the patient needs. And the meals prepared become more low-fat and low-cholesterol because that is what the patient needs, even though other members of the household have no problem with their cholesterol.

What are good and bad ways to ask about relationships?

Bad ways are exclusive and biased. "Do you have a boyfriend? (to a woman)" "Do you have a girlfriend? (to a guy)" "Are you married?" This question privileges heterosexual unions over homosexual unions, since full-fledged gay marriages only exist in one country, the Netherlands, and since legally recognized unions only exist in places like France, Belgium, other European Union countries, Canada, and Vermont. This question privileges the married life over the single life.

Good ways are inclusive and non-biased. "Do you live alone or with someone?" Are you involved with or seeing anyone?" "Are you single, married or partnered?" "What does your partner think about this?" when you don't know the sex/gender of the partner rather than assuming and saying "What does your husband think about this?"

This is also a great strategy when asking about sexual activity. Even in a patient tells you he sleeps only with women or she sleeps only with men, the patient is telling you that in part because that is the answer that a heterosexist society and, odds are, a heterosexist clinician want to hear. If you keep your questioning and statements generic, such as "Next time you are with a sexual partner..." rather than "Next time you are with a guy" sends a strong statement that: (1) you don't care about the sex/gender of your patient's partners; (2) you have a sophisticated and accurate read on human sexuality; and (3) you will be supportive of the patient no matter who their partner.

CONVERSATIONAL RAPPORT

Conversational rapport is rapport that occurs throughout the rest of the encounter. The encounter often proceeds through, though not always: reason for visit*, elaboration of visit**, health history, family history, and social history. This book will now concentrate on reason for visit, elaboration of visit, health history, and social history.

---

* You may know **reason for visit** by the more threatening and counterproductive phrase "chief complaint."

** You may be used to calling **elaboration of visit** as "present illness."

THE REASON FOR VISIT

Once you have ascertained a small sense of who the patient is and where the patient is coming from, it is time to move on and access what brought the patient to see you today.

Good ways to ask

"So tell me what reasons you are here to see me today?"
"What can I do for you today?"
"How can I help you today?"

Less ideal ways to ask

"What's your chief complaint?"
"What problems are you having today?"

ELABORATION OF VISIT

Once the patient has told you the reason(s) for the visit, it is time to follow up on that with the part of the interview called present illness or, better, elaboration.

What's the single worst question you can ask once the patient has provided the reason for visit?

Any closed question of the type: "When did this start?" "Where is the pain located?" "On a scale of 1 to 10 how would you rate the pain?" "Is the pain sharp or dull?" Even though some of these examples are open questions, they focus the patient into a narrow subset of possible responses. Remember if you ask me what my favorite sport is, it is absurd for me to tell you my favorite flavor of ice cream. So if you keep asking me about the quality of my headache, when am I supposed to tell you about the nosebleeds I've also been having. This way of questioning, innocuous as it may seem, can really slow down or derail the diagnosis.

What is the single best question you can ask one the patient has provided the reason for visit?

Any thing like, even if it's a statement, "Tell me more about that" or "Why don't you fill me in on what's been happening. The patient's answer won't take more than a couple of minutes and it will have so many advantages.

1) It will be what anthropologists call thick description, rich with detail.
2) You will get an immediate sense of what is important or troubling to the patient.
3) Sometimes patients present a reason for visit which is not their real reason for visit;
    you will get a quicker sense of this asking this type of statement.
4) Sometimes patients have multiple chief complaints; again you will likely come to this assessment more quickly with this type of questioning.

Then you can zero in with your focused questions, "When did this start?" or "Show me where it hurts?"

Questions to avoid

Unless you are looking for a quick, definitive and specific answer, in the elaboration section it is better to still ask open questions than closed or leading.

"Does the pain occur anywhere else?" rather than "The pain is just in your back?"

"Describe the pain for me." rather than "Is the pain sharp or dull?"

Setting the tone

It is useful to give patient blanket invitations. "If at any time you are uncomfortable or I am hurting you, let me know." "If you have questions at any time, please ask." But it is also useful to give direct invitations. "What questions do you have now?" "Would you like a blanket?"

Now is the time to use umbrella questions.

"What other symptoms do you have?" "What else would you like to tell me about your headaches?" "What concerns you about this?" "What other concerns do you have?" "What else would you like to discuss with me today?"

HEALTH HISTORY

As you move into the health history, the few extra seconds you've spent on rapport might now pay rich dividends for you. The patient will be more relaxed, trusting, forthright with information, and volunteering of information. But you can also use the slightest and most trivial personal information you have garnered to segue into more sensitive questions. Any time you can put a shared connection on a sensitive question, you disarm that question.

Here are some examples that pertain more to the social history. The same approach could be useful for the health history.

When getting to alcohol, you might say, "Ben, you say you're a college student and you like to party. How often do you party?" "Almost every night?" "Wow, I wish I had your stamina. When you party do you consume any alcohol?" This seems far less blunt and invasive then saying out of the blue, "Do you drink alcohol?" Sometimes you have to ask these questions right away and bluntly, but often you can soften or disarm them.

When getting to sexuality and sexual activity, you might say, "Mary, you said you live alone. Are you dating anyone?" "Yes, my boyfriend, Jeff." "Are you sexually active with Jeff?" Or you might say, "Matt, you said you share an apartment with a couple of your college buddies. Are you romantically involved with anyone." "Yes, my boyfriend, Adrian." "Are you sexually active with Adrian? See, inquiring right away and seemingly superficially about residence (or relationships) can help you may these tough questions that less uncomfortable for both you and the patient.

SOCIAL HISTORY

Part of the health history, as you know, is the social history. This part of the interview can produce the most anxiety for both the clinician (especially the novice clinician) and the patient. Here is a protocol for going through the social history which may be helpful to you. Obviously you would customize this for every patient encounter and sometimes parts of the social history will have to be explored during the "reason for visit" or "elaboration," but this protocol makes the social history seamless, matter-of-fact, more clinical, and thus less invasive.

Follow the social history through like this:

daily routine >> leisure >> fitness >> nutrition >> beverages >> caffeine >> alcohol >> recreational drugs >> sexual activity

Starting with a daily routine, which unless the patient is a drug dealer, hit person, or sex worker, can be a fairly innocuous conversation. When people are not working, they have some fun. So what do they do for fun. Now you are talking about their hobbies, and for many that includes exercise, so you have a nice transition to fitness. For those fitness conscious, there is usually an awareness of nutrition, so now you've made the transition to food. From there it is an easy transition to beverages, especially sugared drinks (the patient has a high incidence of caries) and caffeinated. Now you are on beverages, so it's a seamless leap to alcohol. Now you are on substances, so it is a small leap to recreational drugs. (Here, being the good rhetoricians that we now are, we are concerned about language. If you say, "Do you use any illegal or illicit drugs?" in what position does that put your patient? If he or she answers yes, you've just categorized him or her a criminal. This is not the purpose of a health history and physical exam. What does that say about your view of drugs? Though we live in an anti-drug hysteria now, every human society has had its substances of choice, including opium, cocaine, marijuana, nicotine, alcohol, and the like. Coca-Cola once contained wine and coca. FDR's, a U.S. president, grandfather made the Roosevelt family fortune trafficking opium. Middle-class and upper-class citizens can legally sustain their class addiction to Valium or Xanax. Contemporary presidents, Democrat and Republican, have admitted to or have been discovered to have a history of marijuana or cocaine use. Every human culture has its substances of choice. Opium, heroin, marijuana, ecstacy, methamphetamine, nicotine, cocaine, and alcohol will fall out and in favor again in human culture. Any student of human history and human nature can surmise that. Using the word recreational puts you into a partnership with your patient rather than in an adversarial relationship.) Often when we do something we regret or we have something done to us against our will, alcohol or other substances are involved. One thing we regret is unsafe sex and one thing done against our will is sexual assault. So sometimes questions about losing control while under the influence can lead to questions about sexuality. Sometimes you just have to ask about sexuality. But if you use the examples given previously, "You said you live alone, are you seeing anyone?," you can disarm the questions and make them seem less invasive.

SAMPLE REAL PROTOCOL

How would such a protocol play out for real?

Clinician (C): You told me you are an accountant. Let's talk a little more about that.

conversation

C: When you are not being an accountant, what do you like to do for fun?

conversation

C: You said you like to ride your bike. Is that a regular form of exercise for you?

conversation

C: Describe what a typical daily intake of food would be for you?

conversation

C: Do you drink any sugared drinks or caffeinated beverages?

conversation

C: How about using nicotine, either in cigarettes, pipes, cigars or in smokeless tobacco?

conversation

C: Do you use any recreational substances?

conversation

C: Have you ever felt like you lost control of your actions when you use alcohol or cocaine?

conversation

C: You told me you are married. How long have you been married?

conversation

C: Are you sexually active with your wife?

conversation

C: Are you sexually active with any one else?

conversation

C: Two other partners? Were these partners men or women or both?

conversation

C: Did you practice safer sex?

conversation

C: What does safer sex mean to you?

conversation

C: What activities did you engage in with the woman?

conversation

C: What activities did you engage in with the man?

conversation

C: Has your wife had any other sexual partners?

conversation

C: Have these been men or women or both?

and so on

Notice in the sexual history part of the questioning, the clinician did not stop at the comfortable places that our cultural assumptions allow us to.

If you assume a patient married has only one sexual partner, the spouse, or that a patient single has only one sexual partner, the boyfriend/girlfriend, and you ask your questions intimating that assumption or you don't follow up, the patient is prone to play into your assumption. But you don't know the answer; you can only assume the answer that conforms to your worldview and makes you comfortable. That is still not the answer.

If you find out that a male patient has a female wife or girlfriend or that a female patient has a male husband or boyfriend and you find out that your patient has other partners, if you say to the male patient "and when was the last time you were with these other women" or to the female patient "and when was the last time you were with these other men," don't expect the male patient to correct you and say that some of the other partners were men. Similarly, don't expect a correction from a female patient that has been with women. You've just sent a clear and strong signal that you can only process human sexuality in a simple and inaccurate rendering, so the patient does not feel safe enough to correct you or ambitious enough to educate you. And again all you have is your assumption that you have the right answer; you do not know you have the right and complete answer.

You will come across patients who to this point in time have only had sexual encounters with partners of the opposite sex. But some of these patients, more than you might estimate, will have sexual encounters with partner of the same sex in the future. By asking questions in an open, generic fashion—using partner rather than gender specific words—you send a signal that you are sophisticated. The patient will remember you as a sophisticated clinician when he or she has a same-sex encounter in the future and will know that you will treat him or her from a position of caring rather than from a position of heterosexism or homophobia.

Epilogue

Perhaps this handbook has been of some use to you. I hope you have discovered how the questions asked and the words use can really impact the information the patient is able or willing to give you. And that by becoming an amateur rhetorician, it gives you more strategies—more tools in your toolbox—to become and remain a competent, caring clinician who only loses 15% of your patient base each year instead of 33%.

ABOUT THE AUTHOR

Patrick Muller has a master's degree in counselor education. He is a doctoral candidate in higher education. He has taught Rhetoric to first-year college students, communications and histology to dental students, and —as a simulated patient – communication in the physical exam to medical students.

Direct correspondence to:

Patrick Muller
Preventive and Community Dentistry
College of Dentistry
University of Iowa
345 Dental Science North
Iowa City, IA 52240
(319) 335-6594
patrick-muller@uiowa.edu